For Laine and
Lander:
You are always in
my heart

Publication date 2023

ISBN 978-1-59630-118-4

Science & Humanities Press

Saint Charles, MO 63301

Goodbye, Tumor and friends!

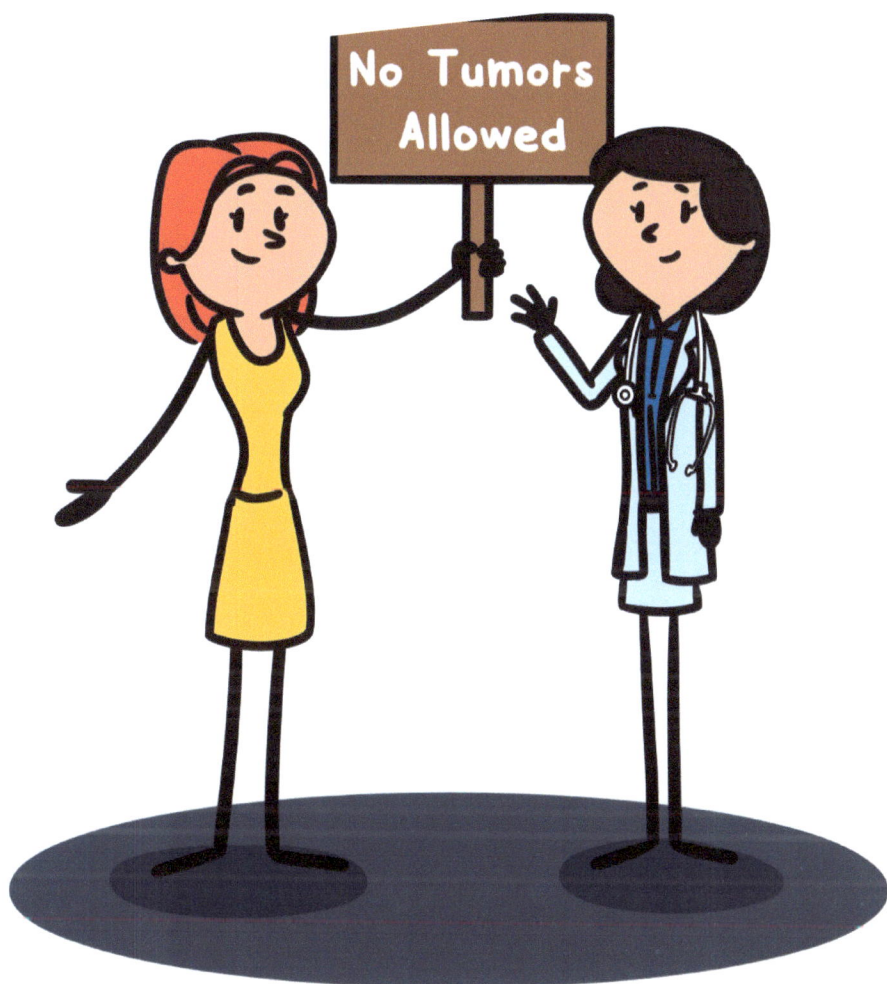

No Tumors Allowed

By Lauren N. Bear
Illustrated by Galihwindu

This is Tumor.

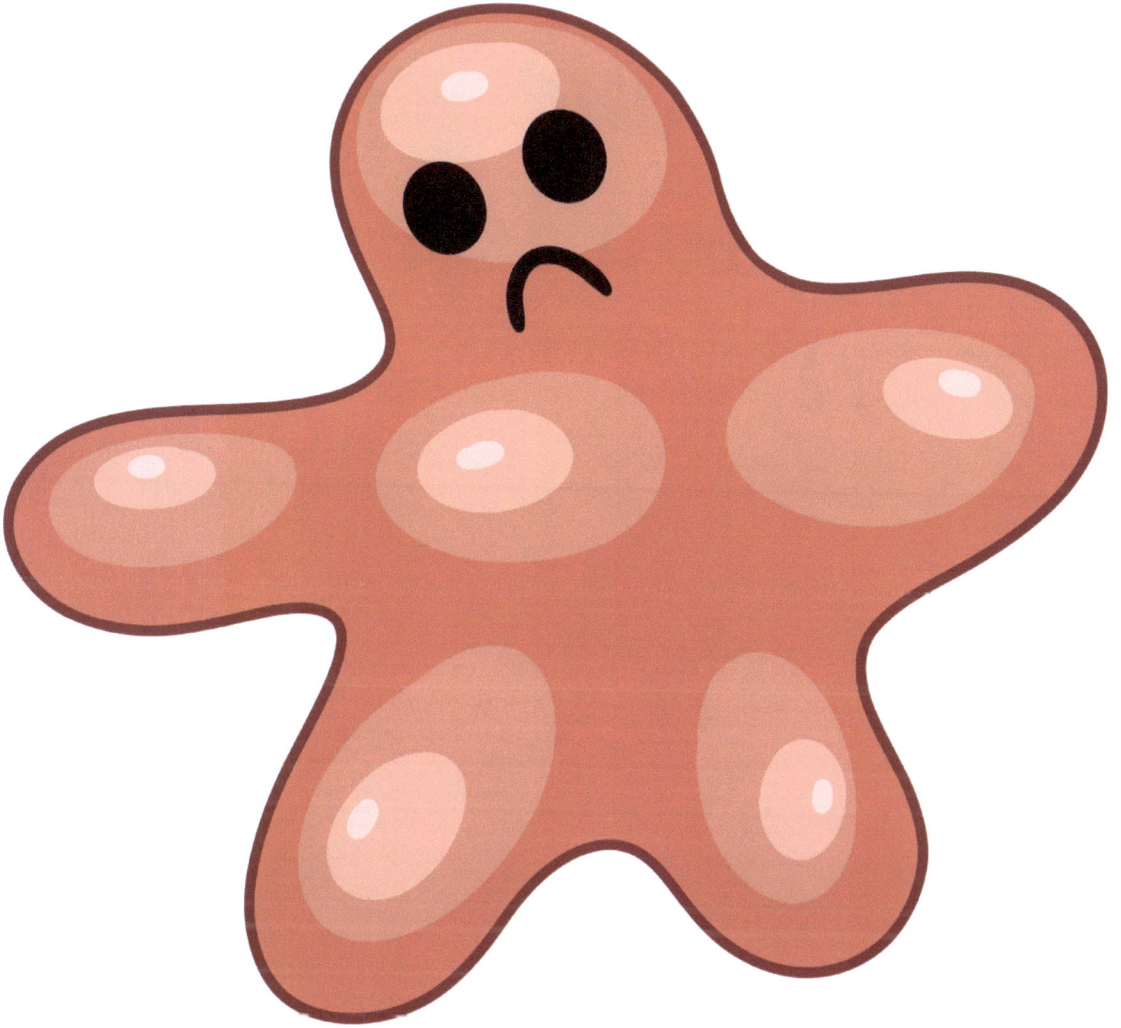

He was growing inside mommy's boobie and wasn't supposed to be there.

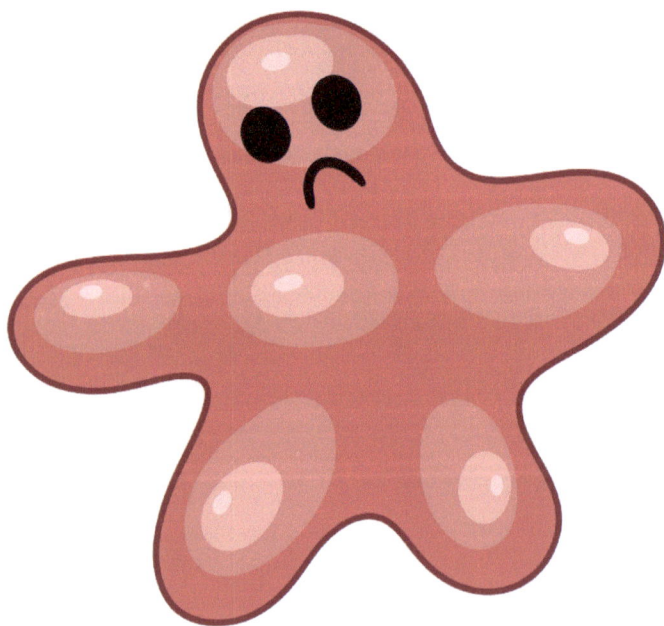

When he grew big enough that mommy and her doctors could notice him, they took him out of her through a little cut on mommy's skin.

This made mommy's boobie ouchy for a while until it healed, just like when you get a cut.

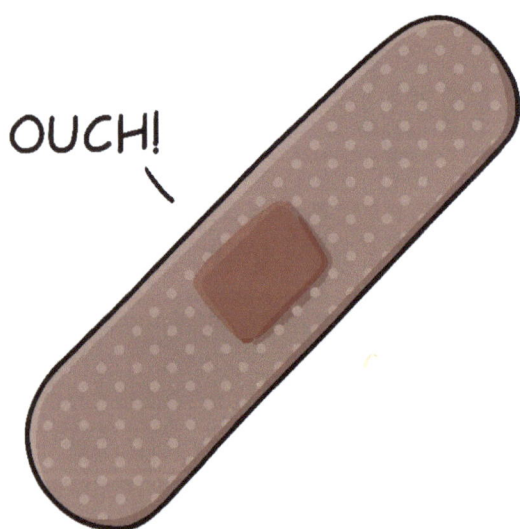

OUCH!

Mommy and her doctors want to make sure Tumor never comes back and none of his friends decide to live in mommy either!

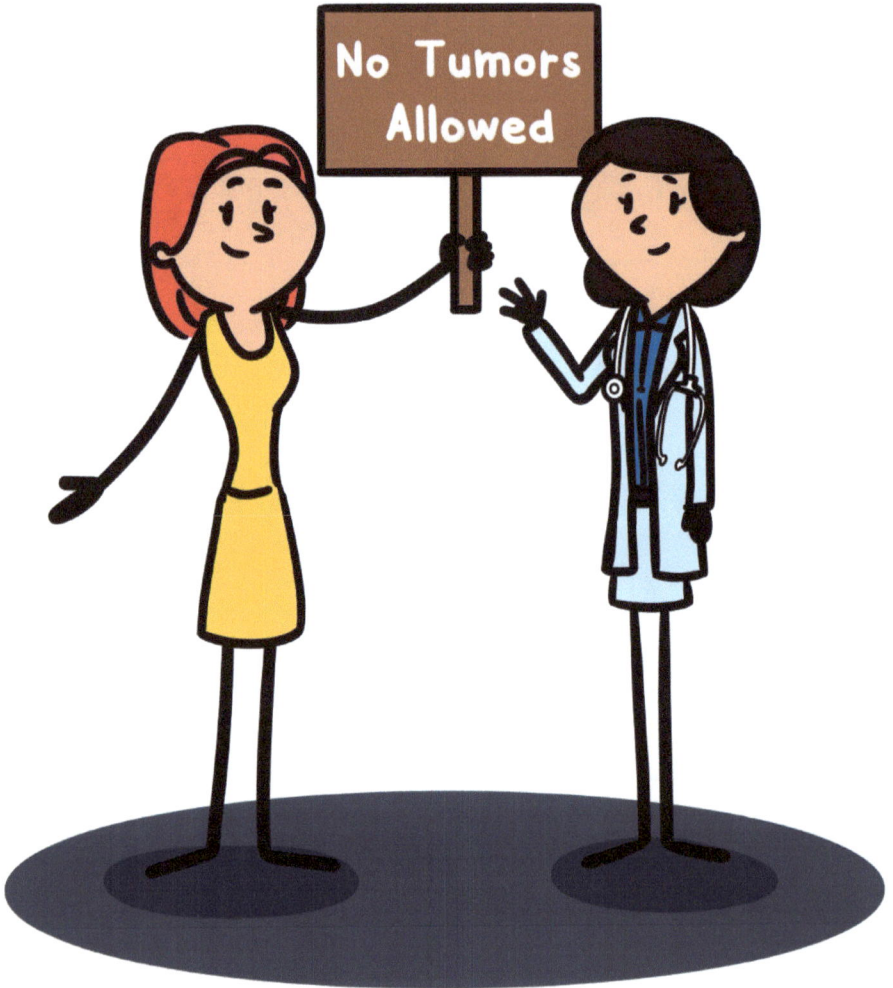

To make sure he doesn't come back and all of his tiny friends are gone, too, mommy's doctors are going to give her a special medicine that tells them to go away!

This is called
Chemo.

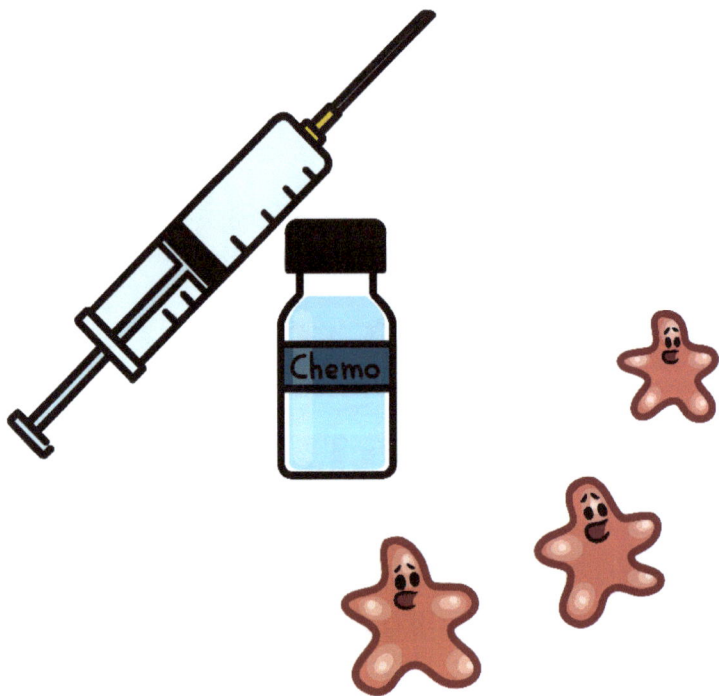

This medicine might make mommy feel sick before she feels better.

It might make her
tired.

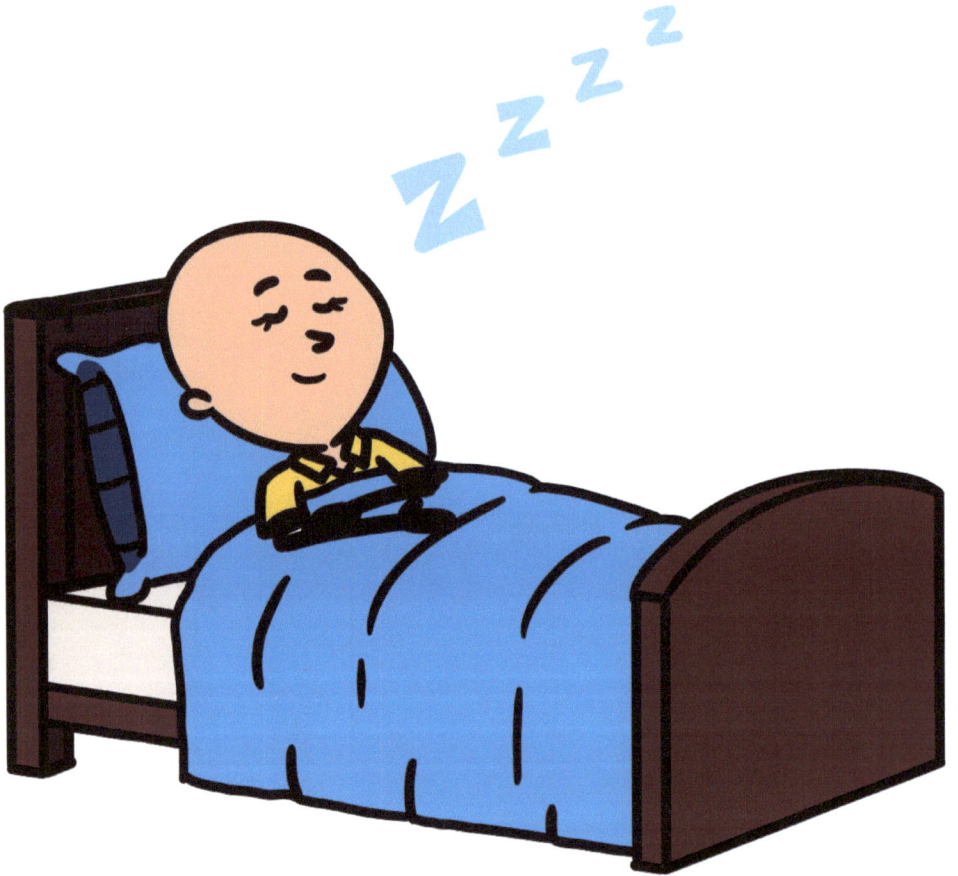

It might make her a little crabby.

It's
a two thumbs
down day!

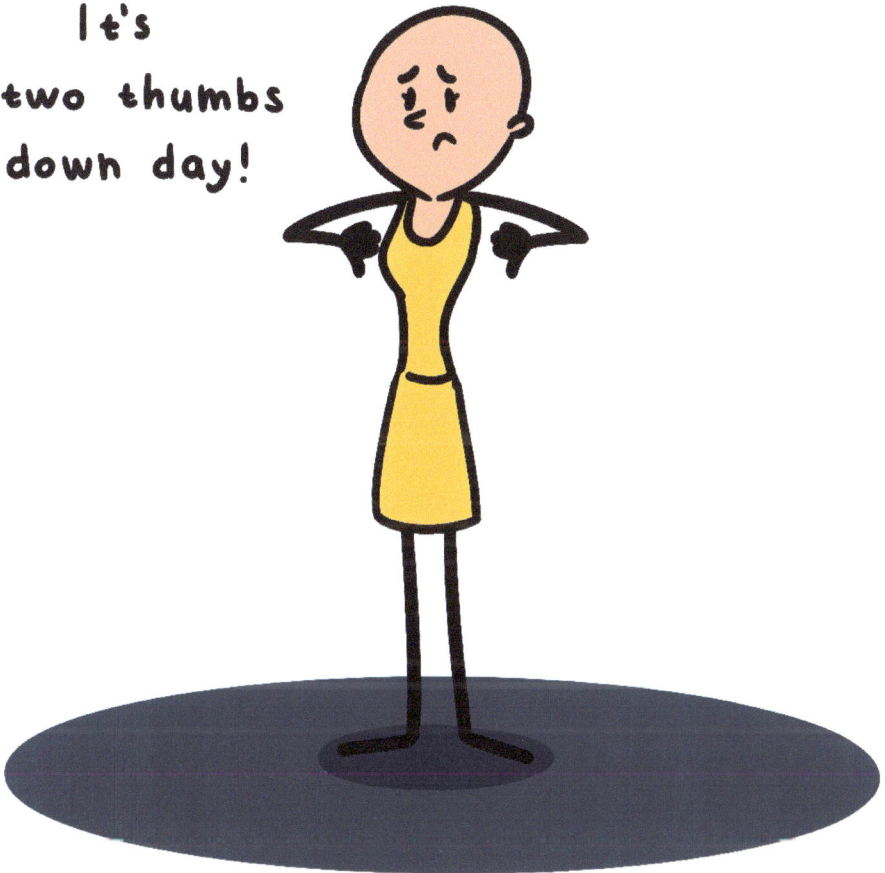

And it's going to make her hair fall out.

Mommy will have fun wigs and hats to wear and will even let you wear some, too!

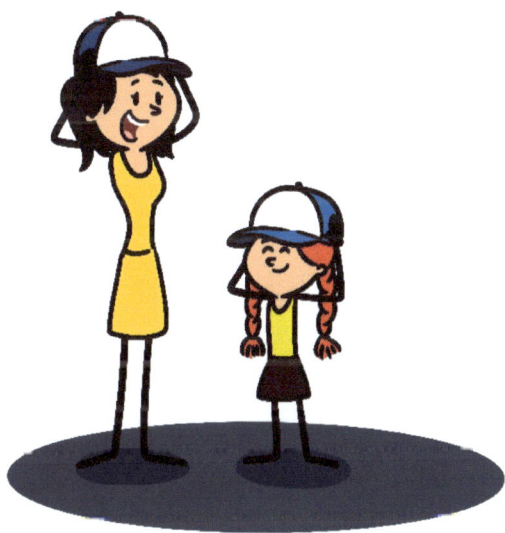

Mommy will need help on some days. You are such a good helper!

She will definitely need big hugs and smiles!

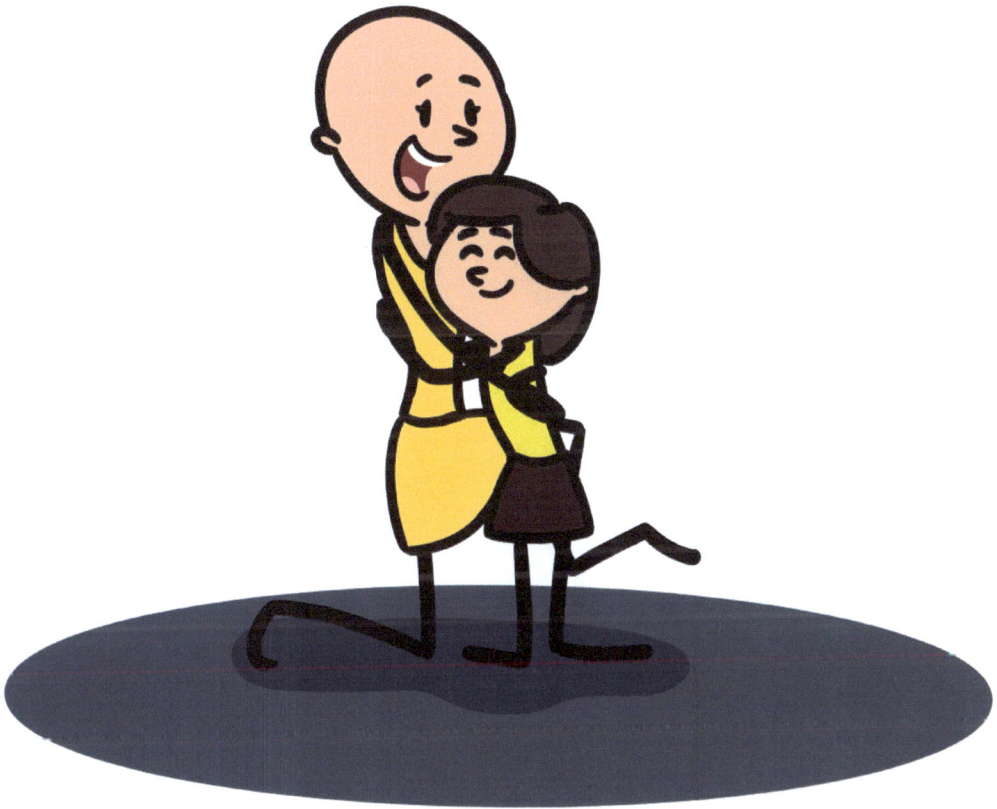

She may need a nap sometimes, too, when you will need to play VERY quietly.

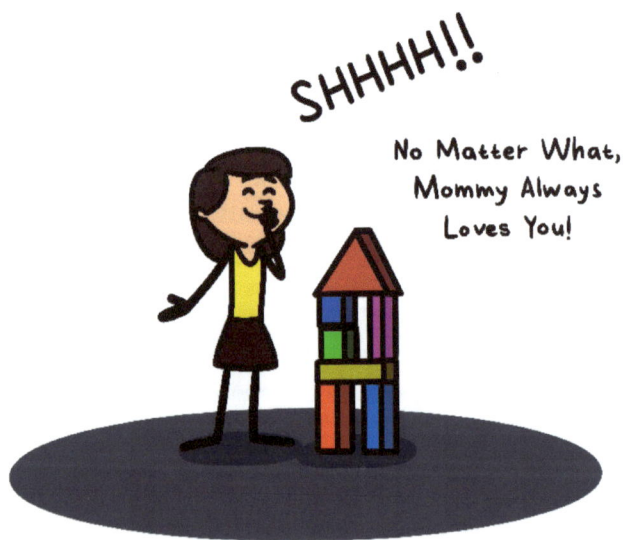

And after mommy is all done with her medicine, which could take a looooonnnnnnnnnggg time...

She will start to feel better again! And her hair will grow back.
It might look different than it used to.

It might be curly.
or a different color.

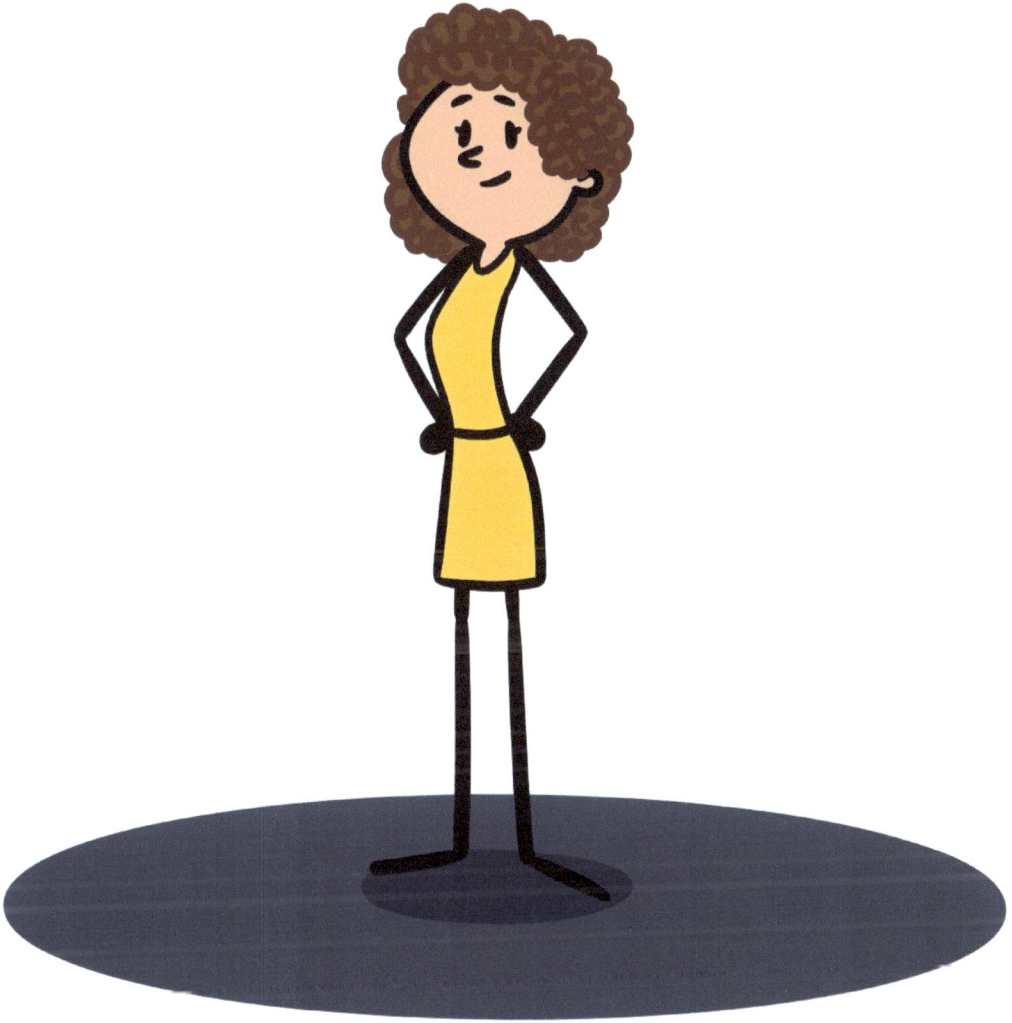

But I'm still your mommy!

And I know Tumor and his friends are gone!

I will go to the doctor a lot to make sure of it!

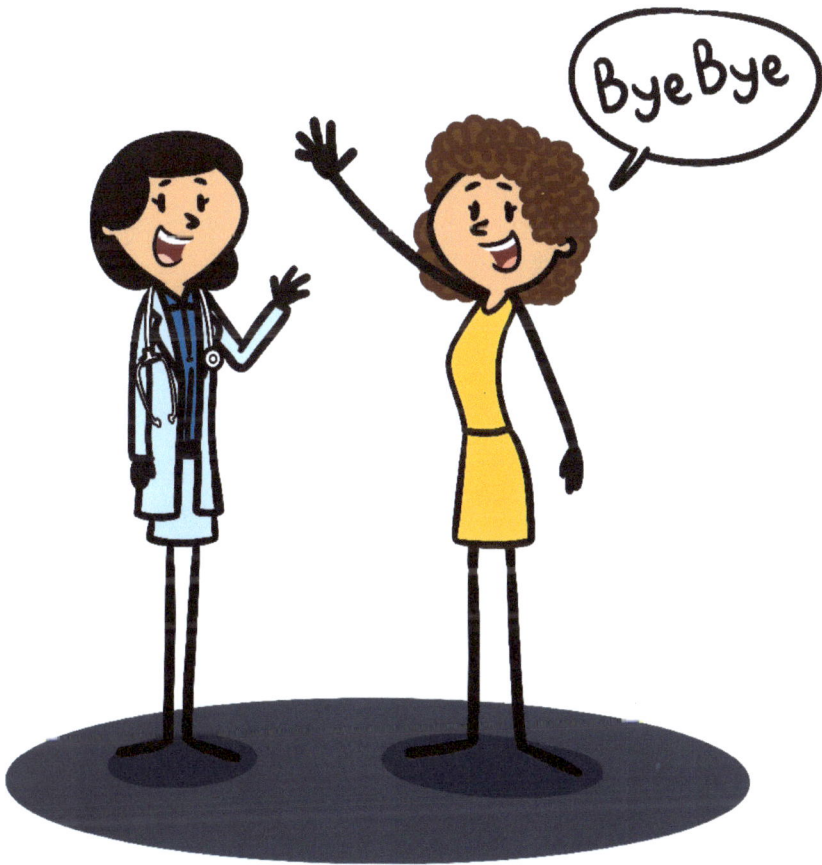

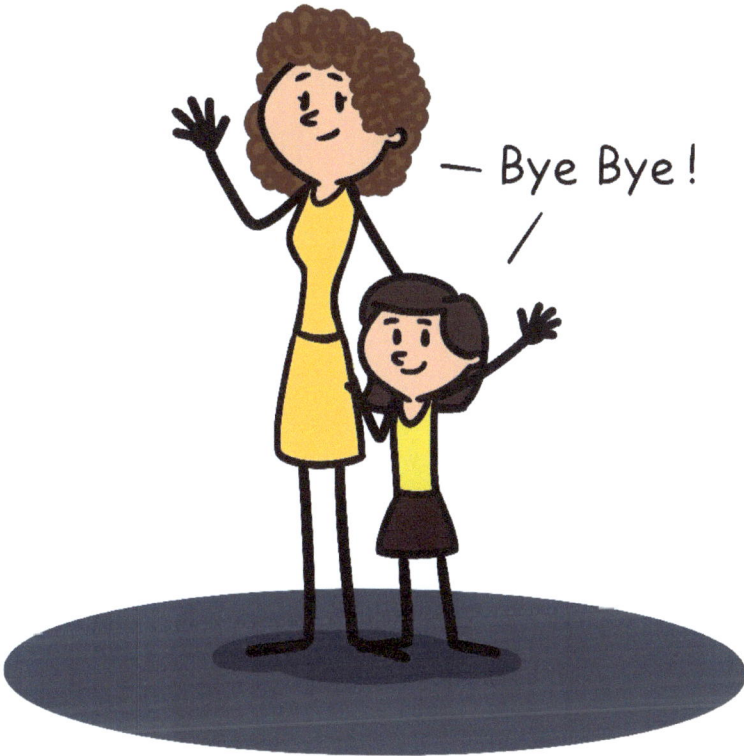

Special Thanks:

To our pediatrician, J. Scott Rogers, for his continued encouragement to publish this book so that other families who need a good resource for their kids would have one available and for his reassurance that I was doing great with my kids even when I felt "two thumbs down" during treatment.

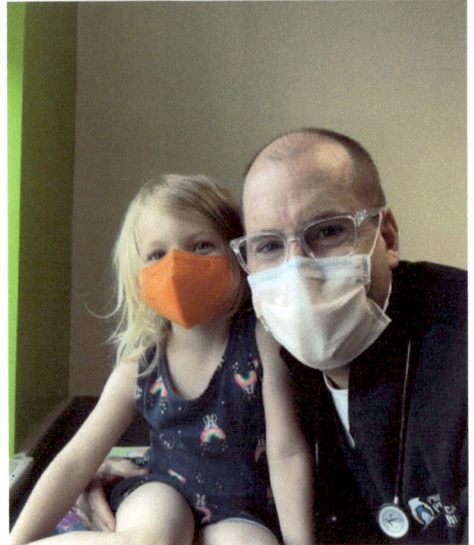

To my oncologists, Anne O'Dea and Melisa Boersma, and the entire team of amazing nurses and technicians at University of Kansas Cancer Center who helped me realize that I can be a strong person without being strong all the time.

About the author:

Lauren Bear was diagnosed with Invasive Lobular Breast Cancer in December 2021 and began chemo in April 2022.

In order to prepare her four-year-old daughter for the side-effects of chemo, she sought out children's books and, when she couldn't find one that provided a simple and age-appropriate message, she wrote her own.

Lauren has been writing short stories and poetry since she was very young, representing her school at a Young Author's Writers' Roundup at the age of 5.

She has since edited books on the side while pursuing her career as a Safety Professional.

This is the first publication of her own work.

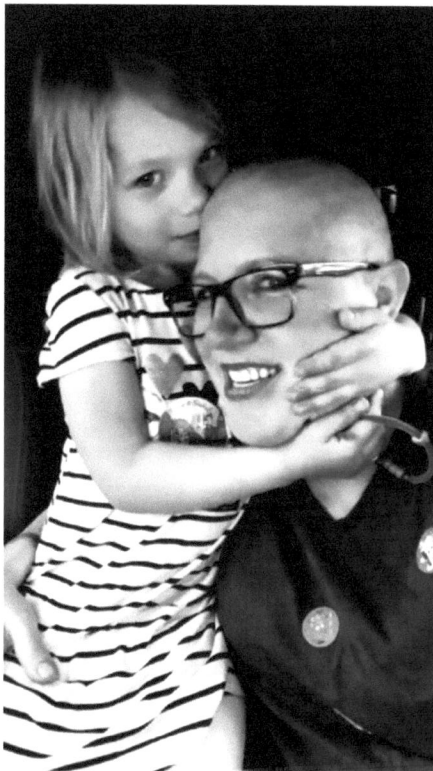

www.ingramcontent.com/pod-product-compliance
Lightning Source LLC
Chambersburg PA
CBHW042109040426
42448CB00002B/192